3/09

PANCREATIC CANCER

Current and Emerging Trends in Detection and Treatment

AMY STERLING CASIL

ROSEN
PUBLISHING®

New York

To my mother, Sterling Sturtevant

Published in 2009 by The Rosen Publishing Group, Inc.
29 East 21st Street, New York, NY 10010

Library of Congress Cataloging-in-Publication Data

Casil, Amy Sterling.
Pancreatic cancer: current and emerging trends in detection and treatment / Amy Sterling Casil.
      p. cm.—(Cancer and modern science)
Includes bibliographical references and index.
ISBN-13: 978-1-4358-5008-8 (library binding)
I. Title.
RC280.P25C473 2008
616.99'437—dc22

                                                              2008025132

Manufactured in the United States of America

On the cover: A colored scanning electron micrograph (SEM) of pancreatic cancer cells joined by a bridge made of cytoplasm (cell fluid). The cells' irregular shape, bumpy nodules, and spiky projections are typical of cancer cells.

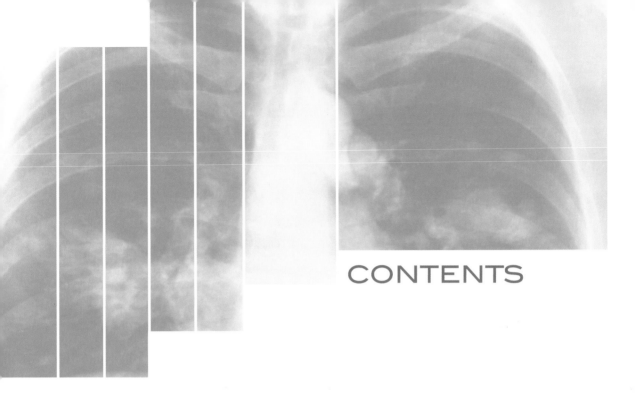

CONTENTS

INTRODUCTION

Next to heart disease, cancer is the second leading cause of death in the United States. Cancer results from abnormal cell growth in which a group of cells begins to grow uncontrollably and invade other tissues, possibly spreading, or metastasizing, to other areas of the body. Cancer of the pancreas is one type of cancer. It occurs when there is an uncontrolled growth of abnormal cells in the pancreas.

Patients with pancreatic cancer receive one of the most serious and grave diagnoses possible, as only 5 percent of patients survive by five years after diagnosis and initial treatment. Among patients with resectable pancreatic cancer (cancers that can be completely surgically removed), there is only a 17 percent survival rate after five years. Unlike breast, lung, and prostate cancers, which have become more curable due to the development of new treatments and diagnostic tools, survival rates of pancreatic cancer have not improved overall during the past twenty-five years.

The high mortality rate for pancreatic cancer, and the difficulty in developing effective new diagnostic and treatment methods, lies in

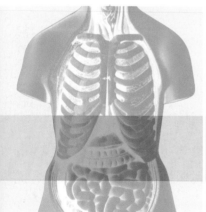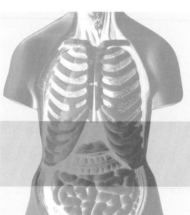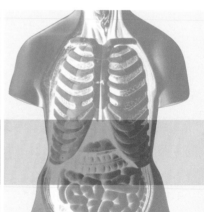

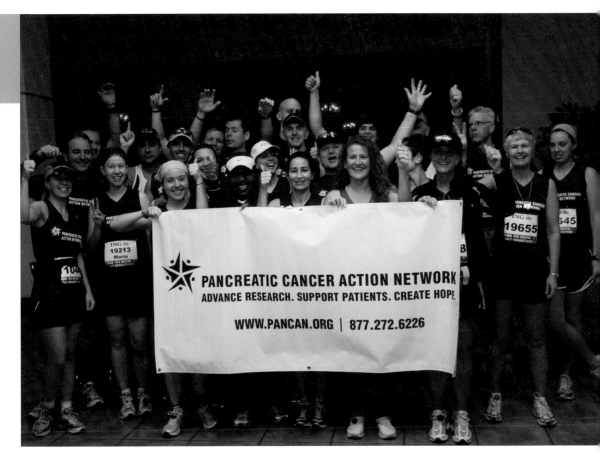

Volunteer events held across the country by organizations like the Pancreatic Cancer Action Network (PanCAN) have raised money for research that may one day result in an effective treatment or cure.

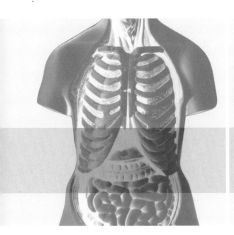
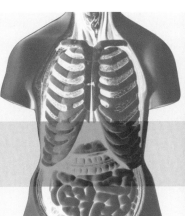
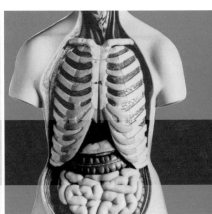

the nature of the disease. Pancreatic cancer is difficult to test for in its early stages, and it spreads very rapidly compared to other cancers. The disease is often very advanced by the time patients experience any symptoms and doctors are alerted to its presence. Most pancreatic cancers are a type of cancer called an adenocarcinoma, which tends to grow rapidly and can spread to other organs in the body.

Eighty-five percent of cancers in the pancreas result from adeno-carcinomas, while the remaining 15 percent are other, rarer forms of cancer. According to the American Cancer Society, about 33,000 new cases of adenocarcinoma of the pancreas (and 3,500 of the rarer types of pancreatic cancer) are diagnosed each year, which represents about 3 percent of all cancers. Although the occurrence of pancreatic cancer is rare compared to a disease like lung cancer, which represents 25 percent of cancers diagnosed each year, pancreatic cancer is the fourth leading cause of cancer deaths in the United States and Canada for both men and women. Overall, the leading causes of cancer deaths are lung cancer, followed by prostate cancer in men, breast cancer in women, and colorectal cancer in both sexes.

Most people are unaware of their pancreas until something goes wrong with it. The pancreas is an organ approximately 6 inches (15 centimeters) in length, located in the upper middle of the abdomen. It is surrounded by the stomach, intestines, liver, and spleen. The head of the pancreas is on the right side of the abdomen. It is connected to the duodenum, the upper end of the small intestine, via a duct (tube). The narrow end of the pancreas, called the tail, extends to the left side of the body. The pancreas makes a variety of enzymes for digestion and hormones including insulin, which regulates the body's use of sugars. Deficiencies in insulin cause diabetes. Development of diabetes is sometimes associated with pancreatic cancer because the growth of the cancer interferes with insulin production.

The risk of pancreatic cancer is increased by a number of factors, but primary risk factors are age (almost 90 percent of patients are older than fifty-five) and tobacco use. As with many cancers, smoking is associated with pancreatic cancer, with smokers being two to three times more likely than nonsmokers to develop the disease, according to the American Cancer Society. Pancreatic cancer is also associated with obesity, a lack of exercise, a diet high in red meat and fat, and, in some cases, a family history of the disease. Sometimes called a "silent killer" because its symptoms are so slow to be recognized, pancreatic cancer represents one of the most serious medical challenges today.

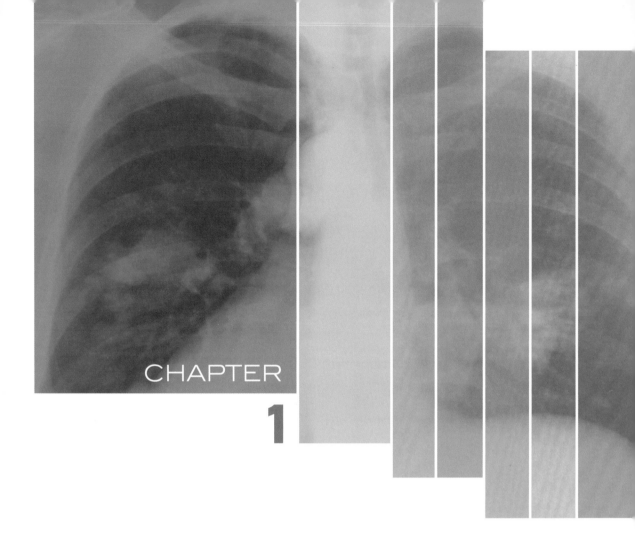

CHAPTER

1

HISTORY OF THE DISEASE

The pancreas was first identified by the Greek physician Herophilus around 300 BCE. Another Greek scientist, Ruphos, named the pancreas, using the Greek words *pan,* meaning "all," and *kreas,* which means "flesh." However, in the English-speaking world, people did not begin to use the word "pancreas" for the organ until about 1570 or 1580.

Alexander the Great, the ancient Greek emperor who conquered much of Europe and Asia during the fourth century BCE, may have been one of the first known victims of pancreatic cancer. It is more likely, how-ever, that he died of acute pancreatitis (an inflammation of the pancreas

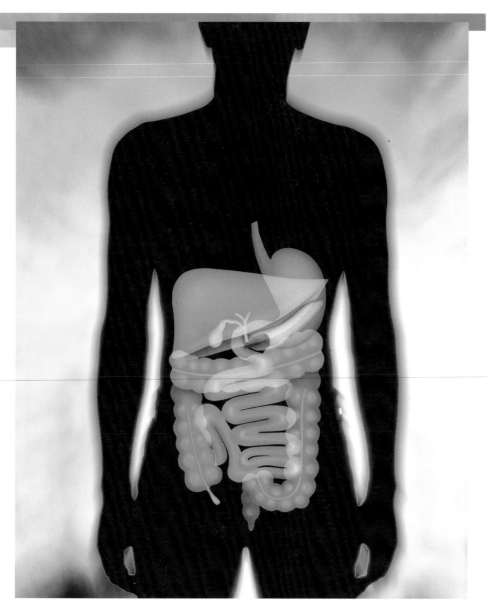

The pancreas is the eggplant-shaped digestive organ lying above the large intestine in the above picture. The pancreas produces hormones, including insulin and gastric juices, that are delivered to the body through the duodenum. Abnormal cell division that starts in the different segments of the pancreas is the cause of pancreatic cancer.

that can be related to pancreatic cancer). Alexander the Great was only thirty-two years old when he died, but he was known for feasting on meat and drinking alcohol excessively. Many pancreatic diseases have been associated with excessive consumption of alcohol as well as red meat.

A POORLY UNDERSTOOD ORGAN

Diseases of the pancreas, such as acute pancreatitis, came to be associated with excessive alcohol consumption or alcoholism. Since alcoholism was often considered a "moral failing," early medical researchers tended to avoid studying diseases of the pancreas.

As a result of the lack of study, the pancreas was long considered one of the most mysterious organs. Reginald de Graaf (1641–1683), a Dutch physician, provided some of the first descriptions of the pancreas and its enzymes. The French physiologist Claude Bernard (1813–1838) described pancreatic secretions and how they aided digestion. He also performed experiments on dogs that helped to identify symptoms such as pale, undigested stools (solid waste) that signified pancreatic cancer or severe pancreatitis in human beings. The next physician to examine diseases of the pancreas was Dr. Reginald Huber Fitz of Massachusetts General Hospital, who in 1889 published the results of his examinations of patients and their autopsies.

A number of ultimately unsuccessful surgical treatments for pancreatic disorders were attempted over the years. Finally, in the 1930s, Dr. Allan Whipple invented the Whipple procedure, a treatment that removed part of the pancreas and surrounding tissue and reconnected the bile ducts, stomach, and small intestines. The Whipple procedure was not easy to perform, and during the 1960s and 1970s, it had a high mortality rate—as many as 25 percent of the patients undergoing the procedure died. Today, however, the Whipple procedure is far more successful, has a far lower mortality rate (less than 5 percent), and is performed for cancer and non-cancer reasons.

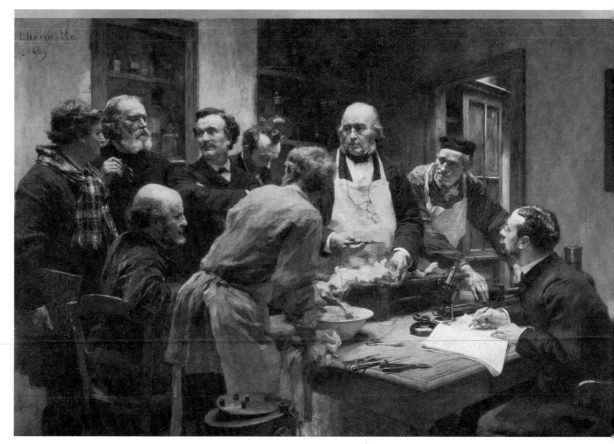

The nineteenth-century French physiologist Claude Bernard lectures his students on anatomy while performing a dissection in this 1889 painting.

LIMITED FUNDING AND RESEARCH

It was not until 1946 that physicians at the Mayo Clinic first described the relationship between family histories and pancreatitis and pancreatic cancer. Although research is ongoing, pancreatic cancer continues to lag behind other cancers in research funding, according to PanCAN, the Pancreatic Cancer Action Network, which is the leading American organization dedicated to fighting pancreatic cancer. Research spending per patient is the lowest of any of the major cancers, at only $1,145 per patient. Only 3 percent of the National Cancer Institute's research budget is spent on pancreatic cancer, according to PanCAN.

Even with limited funding, however, breakthroughs have occurred. In 1952, Drs. M. Comfort and A. Steinberg of the Mayo Clinic first identified a specific genetic component of pancreatic disease. They identified the disease-related gene as cationic trypsinogen, or Try4. This information was key in determining that some people were more susceptible to developing pancreatic cancer due to their family history.

GENE RESEARCH

Later research into all cancers helped to identify oncogenes (genes that cause cancer) and tumor suppressor genes (genes that prevent cancer). In the 1990s, after years of extremely limited research, genes associated with pancreatic cancer went from being among the least understood of all cancer-related genes to the best understood and most researched. The K-ras mutation of genes in cells in the pancreas is associated with 95 percent of the adenocarcinomas of the pancreas (the most common type of pancreatic cancer), and Ras mutations are very common in a variety of cancers, not just pancreatic cancer. Ras mutations are some of the most well-studied and researched oncogenes. K-ras is an abnormal protein, and it is found in the cells of nearly all people diagnosed with pancreatic cancer, even when the disease doesn't run in the family. Correspondingly, inactivation of the p53 gene, a tumor suppressor gene, is associated with the growth of pancreatic cancer. The p53 gene is also an incredibly common tumor suppressor; mutations in p53 genes lead to a variety of adenocarcinomas, including colon and gastric cancers.

In the 1990s, eastern European Jews (also known as Ashkenazi) were discovered to have hereditary risks for several different cancers, including those of the breast, ovary, colon, and pancreas. In 1995, researchers discovered a breast cancer gene called BRCA2, which is also strongly related to the development of pancreatic cancer. Since its discovery, researchers have learned more about the gene's role in cancer. Amazingly, scientists discovered that an ancestor of eastern European Jews, approximately twenty-nine generations or three thousand years ago, developed a defect, or mutation, in the DNA coding for the BRCA2 gene. Today, 1 percent of Jewish people of eastern European heritage have a defective copy of this gene. They are carriers of the gene and thus are at increased risk for developing breast, ovarian, prostate, and pancreatic cancers.

RESEARCH INTO HEREDITY AND BEHAVIOR

In recent years, both heredity and behavior (including health habits) have been found to be connected to pancreatic cancer. In 2004, scientists showed that smoking, which is associated with many cancers, was also strongly associated with the early onset (under age forty) of pancreatic cancer. In 2006, another breakthrough occurred with the discovery of palladin, a gene that caused mutations which in turn caused pancreatic cancer in some families. The palladin gene is located within cells, usually in stress fibers and cell adhesions (connections) to other cells.

The National Familial Pancreas Tumor Registry (NFPTR) is a research registry that was established at Johns Hopkins University in 1994 by Dr. Ralph Hruban. He started the registry so that scientists and doctors could learn more about pancreatic tumors, including why they seem to run in some families. Of special concern with pancreatic cancer is recent research into the reasons why pancreatic cancer is more common among African Americans than among other ethnic or racial groups (other than Ashkenazi or eastern European Jews). According to cancer researchers at Johns Hopkins University, pancreatic cancer is 50 to 90 percent more common among African Americans than among other ethnic populations. Starting in 2005, studies by researchers at the University of California, Irvine, discovered that African Americans had a significantly higher risk of contracting adenocarcinoma. They also had a higher risk of dying from pancreatic cancer than other groups. The researchers recommended increased access to earlier diagnosis and treatment for pancreatic cancer among African Americans.

At the end of three decades of study and research, scientists and physicians have identified some of the common risk factors for pancreatic

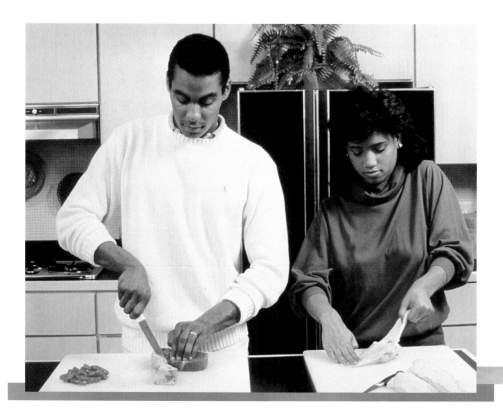

Researchers have determined that African Americans have a significantly higher risk of developing pancreatic cancer. They also have a much higher mortality rate from the disease than other ethnic or racial groups.

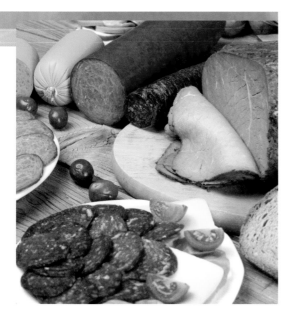

The consumption of red meat has been associated with a higher risk of developing pancreatic cancer. Diet, genetic predisposition, and smoking are the major risk factors for pancreatic cancer.

cancer and have developed a number of treatment options. It has been determined that the largest risk factor is smoking. One 2006 study found that 46 percent of patients with pancreatic cancer had a history of smoking. Also at higher risk are individuals with a family history of pancreatic cancer, people who are significantly overweight or who do not exercise, people with diabetes mellitus or chronic pancreatitis, and, possibly, people who have a high-fat diet and eat a lot of red meat.

EARLY DETECTION STUDIES

The Sol Goldman Pancreatic Cancer Research Center at Johns Hopkins University estimates that 10 percent of pancreatic cancers have a familial or hereditary connection. The National Familial Pancreas Tumor Registry has been established at Johns Hopkins so that scientists and doctors can learn more about pancreatic tumors, including why they seem to run in some families. Studies conducted on Family X, with eighteen members in four generations affected by the disease, led to the discovery of the pancreatic oncogene palladin.

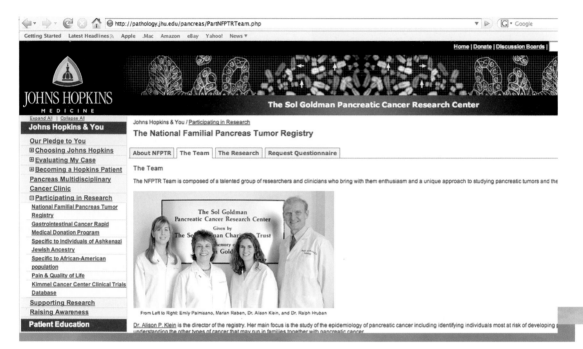

A multidisciplinary team of researchers, physicians, and surgeons at the Sol Goldman Pancreatic Cancer Research Center at Johns Hopkins University (http://pathology. jhu.edu/pancreas/index.php) is leading the fight against pancreatic cancer.

In 2005, *USA Today* reporter Liz Szabo profiled Lori Chappell and her nineteen-year-old son Ryan. Nine members of Ryan's family had died of pancreatic cancer. At age 10, he was diagnosed with diabetes, a disease characterized by problems with insulin production in the pancreas. Ryan's father died of early-onset pancreatic cancer at age thirty-three. Ryan ultimately showed signs of the disease in cancer screenings at the University of Washington, where he was participating in a study to develop new methods of early detection. Because he was participating in the early-detection studies, his mother told Szabo that "Ryan's dad didn't die in vain. Part of him is saving his son."

MYTHS AND FACTS

MYTH I'll feel something is wrong with my pancreas and get it checked out long before a cancerous tumor can grow or spread.

FACT Pancreatic cancer usually spreads quickly and is rarely detected early on. Symptoms may not appear until pancreatic cancer is far advanced and surgical removal is no longer possible. Even when symptoms do begin appearing, such as abdominal pain, lack of appetite, weight loss, and depression, they could be confused with other, less life-threatening ailments.

MYTH Since I have no family history of pancreatic cancer, I don't have to worry about it or make careful lifestyle choices to help prevent it.

FACT Smoking and being overweight are risk factors for pancreatic cancer. In addition, older people, African Americans, and Jewish people of eastern European descent are at higher risk for pancreatic cancer.

MYTH I have a family history of pancreatic cancer, so there's nothing I can do to prevent it.

FACT You can reduce your risk of developing pancreatic cancer by not smoking, maintaining a healthy weight, following a healthy diet, and exercising.

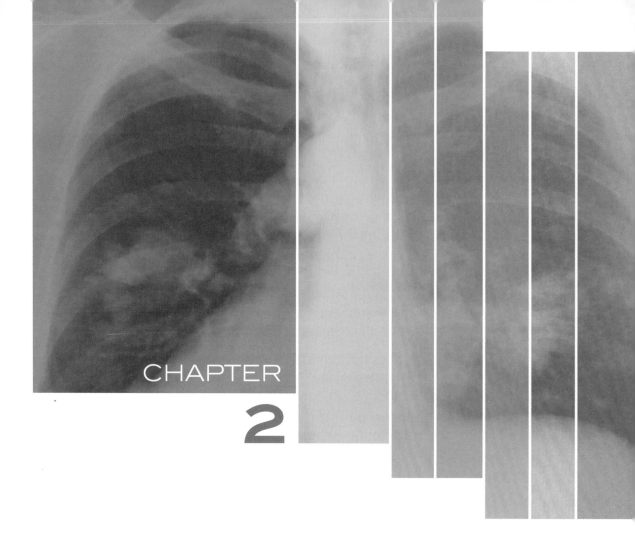

EARLY DETECTION, DIAGNOSIS, AND TREATMENT

Studies of oncogenes, tumor suppressor genes, and heredity have influenced today's pancreatic cancer treatment and intervention. One of the biggest hopes for improvement in survival rates lies in the area of early detection, which has historically been one of the biggest hurdles to overcome in the diagnosis and treatment of pancreatic cancer. The primary cause for the poor survival rates of pancreatic cancer is that it is such a difficult disease to diagnose in its early stages, when it would be more treatable. By the time physicians discover that patients have pancreatic cancer, it is often advanced and it may have metastasized, or spread, beyond the pancreas to other organs.

CURRENT TESTS FOR PANCREATIC CANCER

Current tests for discovering early-onset pancreatic cancer are imperfect, but three tests appear to offer the best chance of finding pancreatic abnormalities. First, doctors can perform an endoscopic ultrasound, in which a specialist inserts a lighted tube through the mouth, down the esophagus, and into the stomach to take a closer look at the pancreas. If that test suggests a problem with the pancreas, then the specialist takes an X-ray after injecting dye into the pancreas's main duct. Injecting the dye can cause an inflammation of the pancreas, or pancreatitis. But if cancer is suspected, the benefits of the test usually outweigh this risk. And if doctors strongly suspect cancer, they might conduct a biopsy, which involves removing a small portion of the pancreas for further testing.

The computed tomography (CT) scan is the most currently used diagnostic tool. Ultrasonography, magnetic resonance imaging (MRI), and two different endoscopic tests may provide additional information. The first of these endoscopic tests, called endoscopic retrograde cholangiopancreatography (ERCP), involves the injection of dye into pancreatic ducts to search for tissue abnormalities. The second, endoscopic ultrasound (EUS), uses sound waves to produce images of the pancreatic ducts instead of the dye and X-ray technique.

Endoscopic procedures are effective because they can detect changes in the ducts of the pancreas. Almost all pancreatic cancers are adenocarcinomas of the ductal epithelium, which is the lining of the duct that connects the pancreas to the intestine. Precancerous lesions of the pancreas, or cancer precursors, are microscopic and can't be

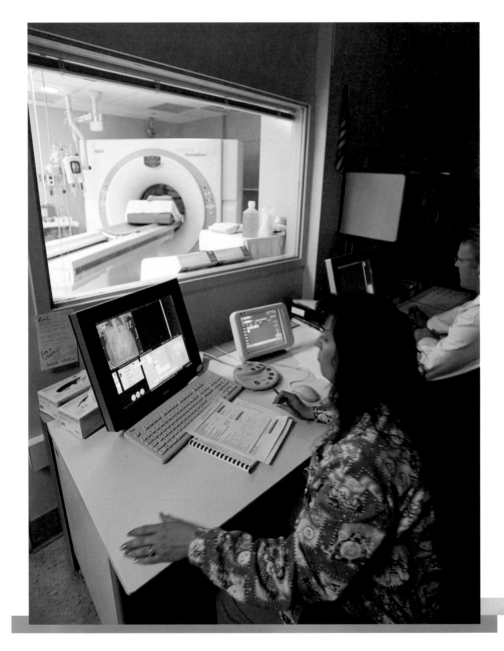

Two technicians operate a computed tomography (CT) scanner. While the patient lies on a table and is examined by the CT scanner, the technicians view the results via computer.

detected without endoscopic tests. According to Lauren O'Malley of Johns Hopkins University, precursor cancerous lesions may be present for years before actual cancer develops. Early diagnostic tests may be used if patients have a number of risk factors, which can include smoking, a family history of pancreatic cancer, a history of diabetes or pancreatitis, or genetic risk factors such as those experienced by Jewish people of eastern European descent or African Americans.

Unfortunately, pancreatic cancer often goes unrecognized and undiagnosed until symptoms appear, which means that the disease is usually far advanced and may have metastasized or spread beyond the pancreas. Jaundice (yellowing of the skin), abdominal pain, and weight loss are classic symptoms of pancreatic cancer. In this case, biopsies are usually performed, which means a surgical removal of tissue from the pancreas, which can then be examined under the microscope by pathologists.

PANCREATIC ANATOMY AND LOCATIONS OF CANCER FORMATION

About 6 inches (15 centimeters) long, the pancreas is located behind the stomach. It attaches to the duodenum, which is the first part of the small intestine. The pancreas is divided into two sections, the "head" and the "tail." The head of the pancreas is the larger part of the organ where it connects to the small intestine or duodenum. The tail of the pancreas is the tapering section extending away from the duodenum and the head.

The tissue of the pancreas is made up of collections of hormone-producing cells called lobules. The majority of the lobules are made up of acinar cells, which are the exocrine-producing cells in the pancreas. The acinar cells form grape-like clusters, which produce the digestive enzymes (proteins) and fluids that the pancreas releases into the small intestine. These enzymes and fluids help us digest food. A smaller number of pancreatic cell clusters form the islets of Langerhans, which

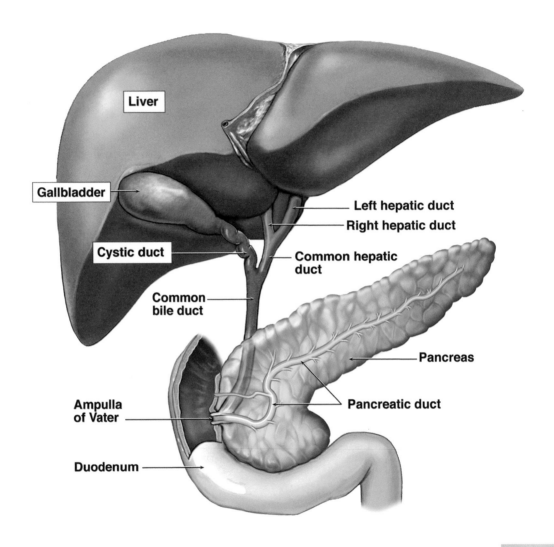

Liver

Gallbladder

Cystic duct

Common
bile duct

Ampulla
of Vater

Duodenum

Left hepatic duct

Right hepatic duct

Common hepatic
duct

Pancreas

Pancreatic duct

When cancer develops in the pancreatic duct or spreads to it from other parts of the pancreas, the disease becomes increasingly difficult to treat.

are endocrine, not exocrine, cells. They produce several hormones, including insulin, which regulates blood sugar levels. The endocrine pancreas secretes four other hormones—glucagons, VIP, gastrin, and somatostatin—that serve other key functions.

More than two-thirds of pancreatic cancers occur in the head of the pancreas, where its duct connects to the duodenum. Because of obstruction of the ducts that carry bile (digestive fluid), symptoms of these cancers often include jaundice and elevated levels of liver enzymes. (Jaundice is a sign of liver infection and disease, and it causes a yellowing of the skin.) Other symptoms of pancreatic cancer related to digestion include pale stools and dark urine.

The other third of pancreatic cancers are tumors in the body and tail of the pancreas. These cancers generally make themselves known through pain and weight loss. Body and tail tumors are much less likely to cause obvious, visible signs and symptoms such as jaundice. Patients may have pain in their abdomen or back, ranging from a dull ache to a severe pain. Tumors in this location usually do not cause symptoms until they have grown quite large. Often, they are discovered as locally advanced disease, with cancer extending to the peritoneum, or the membrane that surrounds the abdominal cavity, and the spleen, the large organ above the stomach that provides valuable immunity against diseases and destroys old red blood cells. Unexplained weight loss of five pounds or more a month or anorexia—the inability or lack of desire to eat—are often symptoms of this type of pancreatic cancer.

Once diagnosed, pancreatic cancers can be categorized as resectable (operable), locally advanced, or metastatic. Resectable pancreatic cancers have not spread beyond an area that surgeons can remove. Locally advanced tumors have spread beyond the pancreas into surrounding tissues and organs. Metastasized cancers are those that have spread from the original tumor (located in the pancreas) to other areas

STAGING FOR PANCREATIC CANCER

Physicians use a system of staging to determine the level of disease and treatment options for all cancers. A specialized system for pancreatic cancer includes seven stages, from cancer *in situ*, or very early cancer, to stage IV, which means that the cancer has spread, or metastasized, throughout the body.

Stage 0 (Tis, N0, M0): The tumor is confined to the top layers of pancreatic duct cells and has not invaded deeper

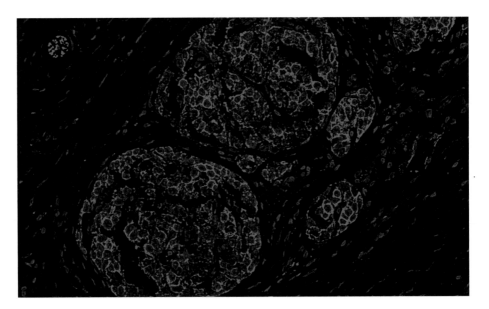

A fluorescence micrograph image of human pancreatic cancer reveals abnormal cell growth, which is indicated by the green areas, that are a kind of protein known as transforming growth factor. This protein causes cancerous cell growth.

tissues. It has not spread outside of the pancreas. These tumors are sometimes referred to as pancreatic carcinoma *in situ* or pancreatic intraepithelial neoplasia III (PanIn III).

Stage IA (T1, N0, M0): The tumor is confined to the pancreas and is less than 2 centimeters (0.79 inches) in size. It has not spread to nearby lymph nodes or distant sites.

Stage IB (T2, N0, M0): The tumor is confined to the pancreas and is larger than 2 cm (0.79 in.) in size. It has not spread to nearby lymph nodes or distant sites.

Stage IIA (T3, N0, M0): The tumor is growing outside the pancreas but not into large blood vessels. It has not spread to nearby lymph nodes or distant sites.

Stage IIB (T1-3, N1, M0): The tumor is either confined to the pancreas or growing outside the pancreas but not into nearby large blood vessels. It has spread to nearby lymph nodes but not distant sites.

Stage III (T4, Any N, M0): The tumor is growing outside the pancreas into nearby large blood vessels. It may or may not have spread to nearby lymph nodes. It has not spread to distant sites.

Stage IV (Any T, Any N, M1): The cancer has spread to distant sites.

and organs of the body. In addition to the bile ducts, the peritoneum, and the spleen, locally advanced tumors often involve the local lymph nodes. The spread of cancer through the lymphatic system is well known, and this is one way in which cancer metastasizes or spreads throughout the body.

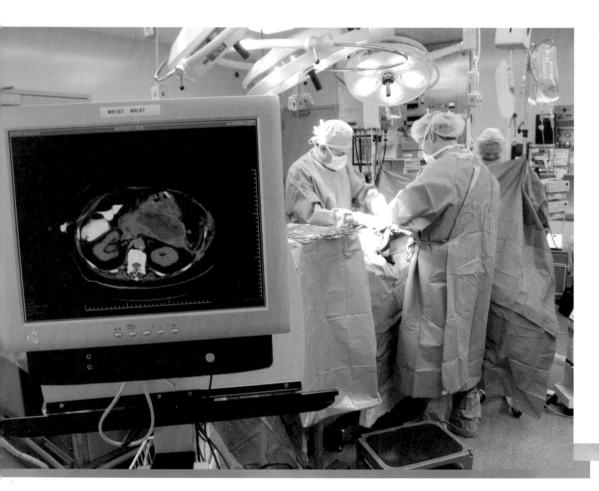

Surgeons perform a cyst-gastrostomy to look for an infected pancreatic pseudo-cyst. Pseudo-cysts usually occur after severe acute pancreatitis, which is a condition related to pancreatic cancer.

CURRENT TREATMENTS
FOR PANCREATIC CANCER

About one in five patients with pancreatic cancer have a resectable tumor, which is one that can be removed surgically. The best treatment for these patients is surgery. If the tumor is not resectable at diagnosis, then the next options are chemotherapy and/or radiation therapy. Even if patients do not have a resectable tumor when they are first diagnosed, chemotherapy, radiation, or a combination of the two may be able to reduce the size of the tumor to the point where it can be surgically removed.

Cancers in the head of the pancreas, which are the most common type, are considered unresectable when cancer has invaded significant blood vessels, called the superior mesenteric artery and vein. Cancers in the tail of the pancreas are unresectable if cancer has invaded the important blood vessels in that area, called the celiac and hepatic arteries. Cancers that have spread beyond the pancreas to other local tissues are not considered resectable, nor are those that have metastasized to other areas of the body.

SURGERY

If the cancer can be removed surgically, then the most common procedure is the Whipple procedure, which was developed by Dr. Allan Whipple in the 1930s. The Whipple procedure remained a dangerous operation into the 1970s, with as high as a 25 percent mortality rate following the operation. Today, however, at major surgical centers such as Johns Hopkins, the Mayo Clinic, UCLA, and USC, experienced surgeons have mortality rates of less than 4 percent, according to the physicians at the Center for Pancreatic and Biliary Diseases at the University of Southern California.

Also called a pancreatoduodenectomy, the Whipple procedure is most commonly used for cancers of the head of the pancreas. It may also be used to treat cancers of the duodenum or small bowel. In the Whipple

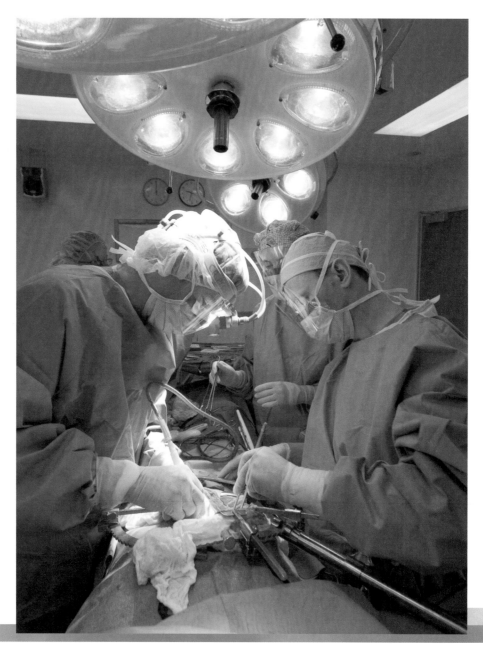

A surgical team performs the Whipple procedure (pancreatoduodenectomy), which involves the removal of the pancreatic head, part of the duodenum, and surrounding tissue to fight pancreatic cancer.

procedure, the surgeon removes the head of the pancreas, most of the duodenum, a portion of the bile duct, and sometimes a portion of the stomach. Afterward, the surgeon reconstructs the digestive tract.

In the less common types of pancreatic cancer located in the body or the tail of the pancreas, another surgical procedure called distal pancreatectomy is used. The tail of the pancreas is removed, usually with the main portion of the organ left intact. A distal pancreatectomy often eliminates the need for surgical reconstruction of the digestive tract.

A total pancreatectomy, or removal of the entire pancreas and many surrounding tissues, sometimes including the spleen, is performed very

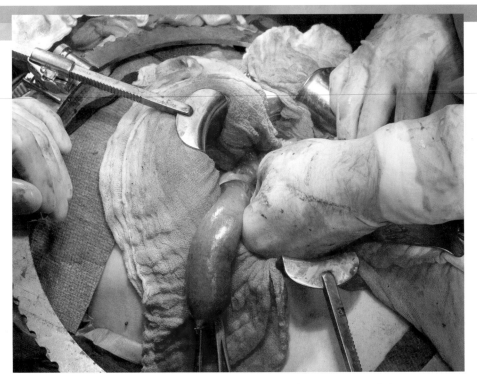

In this photograph taken during a Whipple procedure, a part of the jejunum, which is the central part of the small intestine, is shown.

infrequently because of negative long-term health consequences from the procedure. Occasionally, skilled surgeons may be able to remove portions of blood vessels in the area that ordinarily would cause the cancer to be unresectable. These procedures are rare, however, and depend greatly upon the individual disease and health status of the patient.

Even with all the surgical interventions currently available, pancreatic cancer is a tough opponent. Five-year survival rates for all surgical procedures combined range from 10 to 30 percent. Sometimes, the "cure" may actually do more harm than good. Some recent studies have concluded that chemoradiotherapy (chemotherapy and radiation treatments combined) after surgical resection may actually reduce patients' survival rates. For this reason, current post-surgical treatment focuses on chemotherapy alone.

CHEMOTHERAPY AND RADIATION

Chemotherapy is the use of chemicals to attack cancerous tumors. Gemcitabine is currently the most effective chemotherapy drug for pancreatic cancer, and it may be used alone or in combination with other chemotherapy drugs. For patients whose cancer is advanced and/or inoperable, treatments include radiation in combination with gemcitabine or with other drugs such as fluorouracil (5-FU). Other chemotherapy medications are used for patients with metastatic pancreatic cancer.

Radiation therapy involves the targeted application of radiation to tumors to shrink or kill cells. It is particularly useful for reducing the size of local tumors that cannot be surgically removed. Radiation on its own, however, has not been shown to increase the survival rate for pancreatic cancer. Combined radiation therapy and fluorouracil-based chemotherapy have been shown in recent tests to offer significant survival improvement compared with radiation therapy alone. This course of treatment produced a 40 percent versus a 10 percent survival rate at one year.

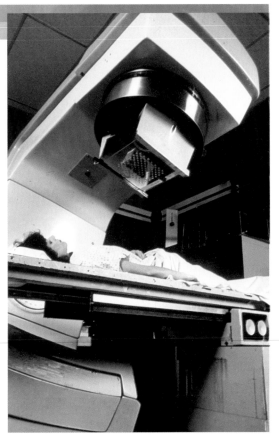

A patient is prepared to receive radiation treatment. Radiation treatments are becoming increasingly sophisticated, as physicians use 3-D imagery and other techniques to target radiation only in cancerous cells, thereby sparing non-cancerous tissue.

Typically, measured doses of radiation of up to 5,000 cGy (centiGray; units of radiation) are administered externally, targeting the cancer cells in the pancreas over a period of six to eight weeks. New methods of radiation treatment are being used in centers across the United States. These include intensity-modulated radiation therapy (IMRT), which delivers a modulated series of radiation doses, and 3-D conformal radiation therapy, which uses computed tomography (CT) scanning to image and reconstruct the tumor and surrounding pancreatic tissue in three dimensions. X-ray technicians can shape multiple radiation beams to the exact contour of the treatment area, which allows a greater amount of normal, non-cancerous tissue to be spared.

At Johns Hopkins University, one of the nation's leading centers for pancreatic treatment, radiologists are using 3-D and 4-D imaging to target cancerous tissue for radiation treatment. This technique helps define the exact extent of tumors, increase the effectiveness of treatment, and minimize damage to healthy tissue in the surrounding areas.

SIDE EFFECTS OF RADIATION AND CHEMOTHERAPY

Many patients fear radiation and chemotherapy because of the side effects of the treatments, which can range from unpleasant to severe. Chemotherapy damages cells that are in the process of division (which is the reason that it can affect cancer cells, which divide and grow rapidly).

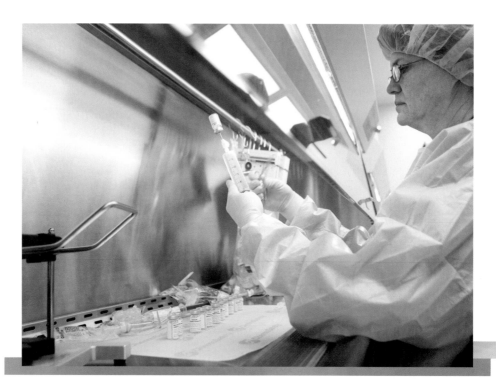

Cyndee Thomas, a pharmacy technician at the North Idaho Cancer Center in Coeur d'Alene, Idaho, mixes chemotherapy medications. The facility takes part in clinical research trials of experimental cancer drugs.

Many chemotherapy medications also affect the body's healthy tissues, particularly ones that are growing rapidly.

Common side effects of chemotherapy vary from drug to drug. Side effects for the common pancreatic cancer chemotherapy drug 5-FU include fatigue, decreased bone marrow function, loss of appetite, a sore mouth (because mucous membranes are being destroyed by the drug in addition to cancer), diarrhea, and nausea. Gemcitabine, the other common chemotherapy treatment, can cause fatigue, decreased bone marrow function, hair loss, soreness in the palms of the hands and soles of the feet, and digestive distress and diarrhea. Skin problems such as burns and rashes, fatigue, nausea and loss of appetite, and hair loss are the most common side effects of radiation therapy.

Side effects always vary from patient to patient, and most of the problems result from the destruction of cells, which is part of the process of destroying the cancer. Overall, the benefits of treatment outweigh the problems of chemotherapy or radiation treatments.

PALLIATIVE CARE

Because the prognosis for pancreatic cancer is poor, with low five-year survival rates, palliative care is a high priority for physicians. The goal of palliative care is to improve the quality of life for severely ill patients. Palliative care, by definition, is not treatment that strives for a cure. It is treatment through chemotherapy, radiation, and other methods that relieves patients' pain and suffering and improves their quality of life. Palliative care is often combined with hospice care and treatment for depression.

Treatments involving palliative care may include surgery to stop nerve pain in the area of tumors, as well as chemotherapy and radiation to shrink tumors to reduce pain and suffering. These measures may be taken even when physicians know that a cure cannot be obtained.

TEN GREAT QUESTIONS
TO ASK YOUR DOCTOR

1. What can I do to help prevent pancreatic cancer, or at least reduce my risk of getting it?

2. If I don't have a family history of pancreatic cancer, how worried should I be about developing it? How worried should I be if I do have a family history of the disease?

3. What is the best available, most successful treatment option for pancreatic cancer?

4. How can I improve my chances of detecting pancreatic cancer early?

5. Is there any test I can take to learn if I am genetically disposed to pancreatic cancer?

6. What are the tell-tale signs and symptoms of pancreatic cancer?

7. What is the first step to take after receiving a diagnosis of pancreatic cancer?

8. A family member has pancreatic cancer. How do we learn if the cancer has spread elsewhere in the body?

9. How should my family member prepare for surgery, chemotherapy, and/or radiation?

10. What are some of the clinical trials going on right now, and would you recommend that my family member get involved in any? What are the risks of clinical trials, and what are the possible benefits?

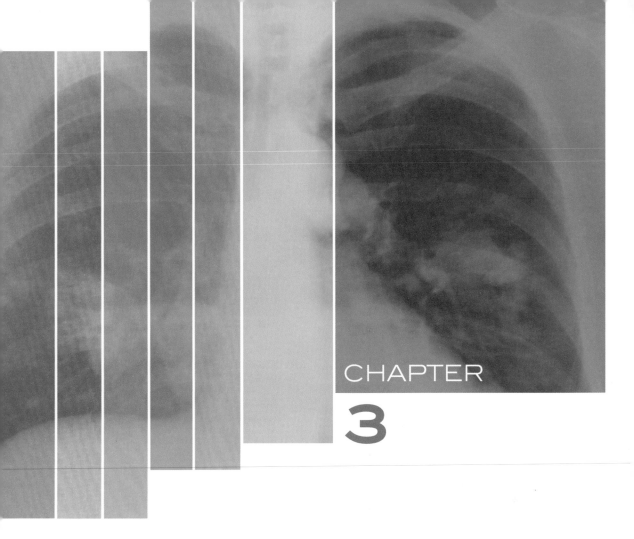

CURRENT RESEARCH

Because pancreatic cancer is so often a "silent" disease, it is frequently very advanced by the time patients experience symptoms. The combination of the difficulty in treating the disease and poor survival rates meant that, in the past, other, more readily diagnosed and treated cancers received greater levels of research, funding, attention, and higher rates of treatment development. These cancers, such as those of the breast, colon, and prostate, are all much more common in occurrence than pancreatic cancer. Yet, rates of pancreatic cancer deaths are much higher.

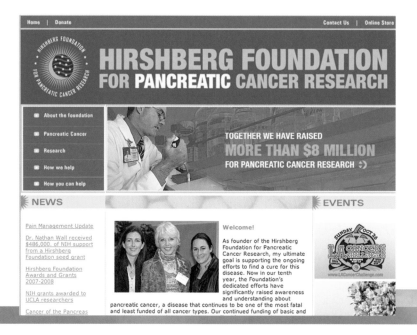

Pancreatic cancer research is led by privately funded cancer research organizations such as the Hirshberg Foundation for Pancreatic Research (www.pancreatic.org), which helps to support research at UCLA and other medical facilities.

Interest in pancreatic cancer is on the rise among researchers, however. Advocacy organizations such as the Hirshberg Foundation for Pancreatic Research, the Pancreatic Cancer Action Network, and the Sol Goldman Pancreatic Cancer Research Center at Johns Hopkins have drawn attention to potential research and clinical studies. According to the National Cancer Institute, which is part of the National Institutes of Health, the Institute's spending on pancreatic cancer research grew from $21.8 million to $74.2 million since 2001, and the number of investigators receiving grants increased 171 percent. Since 2000, the number of medical researchers working with pancreatic cancer has increased from thirty-two to more than ninety nationwide.

Current research is divided between investigation into the causes of pancreatic cancer, early detection of the disease, and potential treatments. Successful research is being conducted into gene therapy and vaccines. These are not meant to cure the cancer but help slow its progress. Research into the causes and risk factors for pancreatic cancer also continues. A recent study sponsored by the National Cancer Institute indicates that people who eat more fruits and vegetables, and less fat and red meat, experience a lower incidence of pancreatic cancer, even if they possess higher risk factors such as a family history or smoking.

MAKING PROGRESS

According to the National Cancer Institute, an estimated 37,130 people will be diagnosed with pancreatic cancer and an estimated 33,370 deaths will occur in 2008. The total number of pancreatic cancer cases and deaths has increased since 2003, but the rate of pancreatic cancer deaths as compared to new diagnoses has slowed between 2006 and 2007. Because researchers have recognized that African Americans suffer higher rates of pancreatic cancer than other groups, some research studies and recommended screening procedures have had an impact. National Cancer Institute statistics show that, while rates of pancreatic cancer deaths among African Americans are still disproportionately high, they are decreasing.

Setting priorities for research studies has helped to make progress against the disease. In 2001, the National Cancer Institute prioritized the development of expanded training and career development efforts and the establishment of "centers of excellence." Today, Specialized Programs for Research Excellence, or SPOREs, for pancreatic cancer research are located at the Mayo Clinic, the University of Texas M.D. Anderson Cancer Center, and the University of Alabama-Birmingham Pancreatic SPORE Program. Overall, through SPORE and other funded research programs, the greatest focus is on the highest area of needs: research into the causes, effects, and potential cures of adeno-carcinoma, the fastest-growing, most serious, and most common type of pancreatic cancer.

In February 2007, a group of researchers at the University of Michigan Medical Center discovered the small number of cells in pancreatic cancer that are capable of fueling tumor growth. This discovery was the first identification of cancer stem cells in pancreatic tumors. Having identified these stem cells, researchers can now try to develop drugs that will target and kill these cells. Many of the researchers believe that other cancer treatments often fail because they do not attack the cancer stem cells that cause tumor growth.

ANALYZING RISK FACTORS

Another important focus of current research into pancreatic cancer is identifying risk factors for the disease and developing models for intervention and prevention. One example is a recent study funded by the National Cancer Institute at Virginia Polytechnic Institute. The five-year study has developed a lifestyle modification program in the areas of diet and exercise for patients with the pancreatic cancer risk factors of obesity and low physical activity. Two groups of patients participating in guided fitness and exercise programs are being studied to determine the impact of fitness, exercise, and lifestyle enhancement programs in preventing the occurrence of pancreatic cancer.

Few large-scale studies of risk factors for pancreatic cancer have been conducted due to the rapid progress and high mortality rate of the disease. Yet, the Center for Health Studies in Seattle, Washington, is nearing the completion of a five-year study on more than 1,400 patients with the goal of investigating the relationship between pancreatic cancer risk and diabetes, diet, insulin resistance, non-steroidal anti-inflammatory drugs (NSAIDS), and direct and indirect exposure to tobacco and pancreatic cancer.

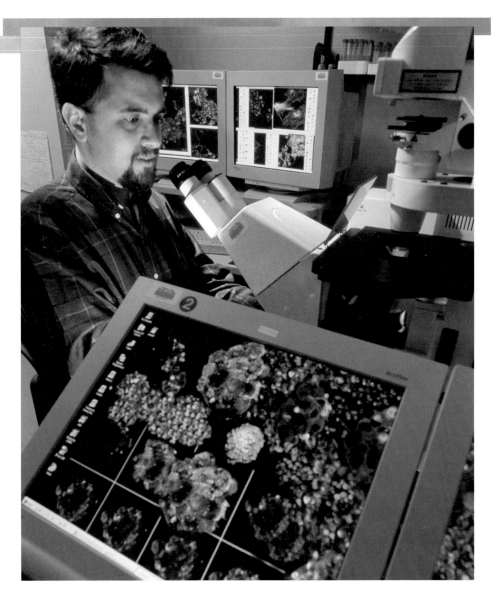

Research into other health conditions assists the fight against pancreatic cancer. Here, a researcher uses a laser scanning microscope to view pancreatic beta cells as part of a diabetes study at the National Institute for Digestive and Kidney Diseases at the National Institutes of Health in Bethesda, Maryland.

An extended research study of existing pancreatic cancer patients at the University of Texas M.D. Anderson Cancer Center is evaluating the impact of diets and lifestyle habits that include high levels of red meat consumption combined with histories of tobacco smoking. Pilot studies have already determined a connection between metabolic genes and a specific DNA repair gene among patients who have a genetic

A FAMOUS FAMILY CONFRONTS PANCREATIC CANCER

Former U.S. president Jimmy Carter has lost four relatives to pancreatic cancer. The Carter family is not only the best known but is also one of the most devastated families as a result of the disease. In 2007, Carter told the *New York Times*, "We started out a long time ago with my father dying of pancreatic cancer. One by one, both my sisters and brother died of pancreatic cancer." In addition to their personal tragedy, the Carters have participated in the National Familial Pancreas Tumor Registry and other programs to discover the hereditary components of pancreatic cancer.

Carter said doctors had offered various theories about what had caused so much disease in his family. "Nobody knew," he said. "They thought my family [who had all worked in farming] might have imbibed some kind of poison, a pesticide. Back in the olden days, the federal government didn't care what kind of poison you used." However, Carter also told the *New York Times* that all of his family members who had contracted pancreatic cancer had also smoked, while he had not. This could explain why he has not contracted the disease and has reached his eighties in excellent health.

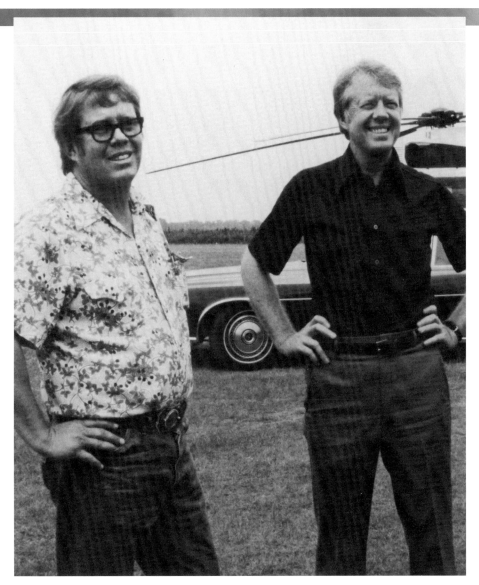

Former U.S. president Jimmy Carter (right) and his brother, Billy, share an informal family reunion on St. Simon's Island, Georgia, in 1977. Billy Carter died of pancreatic cancer in 1988.

susceptibility to pancreatic cancer and have the risk factors of high red meat consumption and/or smoking.

STUDIES OF GENETIC FACTORS AND STEM CELLS

Because the most common type of pancreatic cancer, adeno-carcinoma, has been found to be more resistant to chemotherapy than many other types of cancer, studies have also focused upon ways to better understand the cell function and drug resistance properties of pancreatic cancer cells. A five-year study funded at Johns Hopkins University is focusing on a recently discovered cancer-recurrence gene called NAC-1, with the hope that more will be learned about the role of NAC-1 in tumor progression. Johns Hopkins researchers also hope to discover the molecular foundation for the NAC-1 gene, which will assist in the development of more effective drug therapies to suppress tumor growth.

The 2007 discovery of pancreatic cancer stem cells helped researchers to better understand the rapid growth and aggressiveness of pancreatic cancer. Previous research into breast cancer stem cells helped to identify cell proteins that also characterized pancreatic cancer stem cells. Although the fast-growing and drug-resistant cancer stem cells seem to be a tough opponent right now, researcher Dr. J. Milton Jessup of the National Cancer Institute said, "The study shows that it is possible to isolate the pancreatic cancer stem cell in order to investigate its properties, determine its weaknesses, and then develop therapies that target this cell." Jessup also noted that although cancer stem cells appear to be relatively resistant to therapy, "these cells may prove to be the Achilles heel of the cancer" (as quoted by the American Cancer Society).

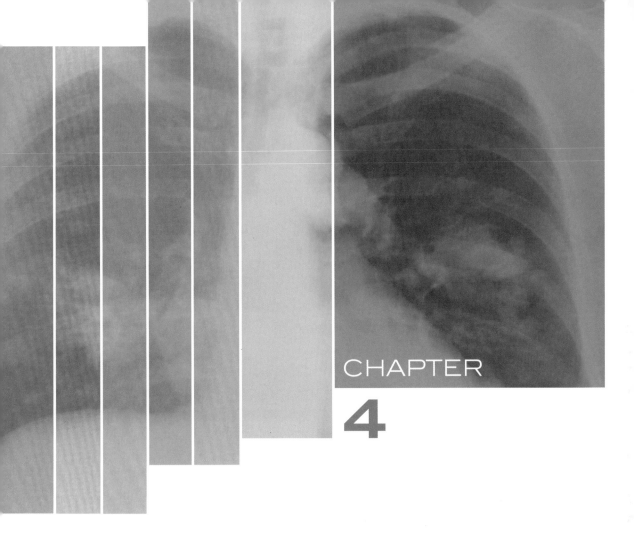

NEW STUDIES AND
FUTURE TREATMENTS

Pancreatic cancer (as well as many other cancers) has been shown to be related to an immune system response. Much current research is focused upon potential methods of suppressing immune system responses that appear to cause growth of the cancer, as well as on increasing immune responses that can fight the cancer. Early detection of the disease through improved screening methods is also a high priority for physicians and scientists. An ideal pancreatic cancer-screening test would be safe, inexpensive, and highly accurate.

CUTTING-EDGE RESEARCH

Research continues into discovering which patients have a genetic tendency toward developing pancreatic cancer. Cancer research in general has led scientists to discovery of the tumor-causing genes BRCA2, p16, and HNPCC (hereditary non-polyposis colon cancer, which can lead to a genetic type of colo-rectal cancer and to pancreatic cancer). Researchers are now seeking answers to how these genes may be altered in patients with pancreatic cancer and who do not seem to have a family history of pancreatic cancer but nevertheless possess these genes.

Scientists have also determined that additional changes in the DNA and other cellular molecules in the pancreas cause pancreatic cancer that is not related to heredity or genetics. Smoking, a diet high in fat and red meat, and advanced age are all factors that can alter DNA in such a way as to make pancreatic cancer possible. Pancreatic cancer researchers continue to identify these specific changes in DNA and other molecules. Within the next few years, the research will lead to new, specific, and sensitive screening tests, including serial analysis of gene expression (SAGE) tests that may be able to identify pancreatic cancer at a stage that is even earlier than it can be currently detected with sensitive diagnostic imaging techniques. The first group of patients who will be able to benefit from the new DNA and other molecular-based tests will be those with a combination of serious risk factors or a family history of the disease.

According to the American Cancer Society, researchers are also studying growth factor receptors and inhibitors. Cancer cells, including pancreatic cancer, have molecules on their surfaces that help them to grow. Some of these are called growth factor receptors. One influential receptor is epidermal growth factor receptor (EGFR). Chemotherapy drugs targeting EGFR are now being studied, including erlotinib (Tarceva),

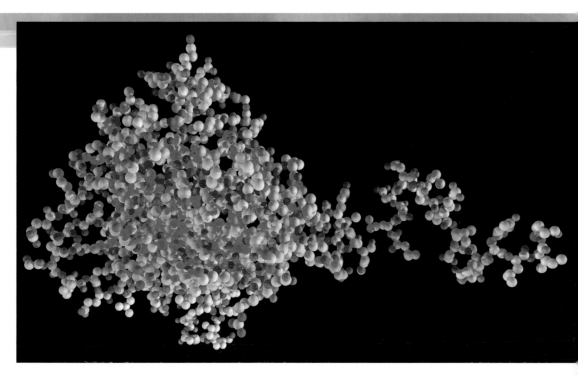

A model of the protein molecule called the epidermal growth factor receptor (EGFR) is shown here. Mutations involving EGFR have been linked to pancreatic cancer and other cancers. EGFR inhibitors have been developed to target these cancer-causing molecules.

that have been approved for use with the established drug gemcitabine in the United States and Canada. Other drugs are still in clinical trials that could prove more effective, such as cetuximab (Erbitux).

Cancer cells also depend upon encouraging new blood vessels to grow to feed tumor growth and development. This is a process called angiogenesis. To block angiogenesis and prevent blood from reaching the tumor, scientists are developing anti-angiogenesis drugs. These are being studied in clinical trials and may be used in patients with pancreatic cancer. Some early studies have found that the anti-angiogenesis drug bevacizumab, also known as Avastin, may help fight pancreatic cancer when combined with gemcitabine. Larger studies are now under way to figure out how active this drug is. More anti-angiogenesis drugs are also being studied.

Many drugs targeting other aspects of cancer cells are also being studied for use in pancreatic cancer. Drugs that target the action of farnesyl transferase, an enzyme that is thought to stimulate the growth of many cancers, are now being tested.

CANCER VACCINES

One hope for future treatment lies in the area of cancer vaccines. These are designed to try to stimulate the body's own immune system to fight cancer. The immune system naturally attacks foreign cells that are invading the body, such as bacteria and viruses. Cancer cells can also be recognized by the body as foreign because they are chemically different from normal cells. However, the development of cancer vaccines is much more challenging than the development of vaccines to combat infectious diseases. This is because cancer cells develop from normal body cells, making them much harder for the immune system to spot and differentiate from healthy cells.

Pancreatic cancer vaccines are designed to recognize abnormal proteins made by pancreatic cancer cells, which include the K-ras gene protein. The vaccine will then "lock on" to the cancer cells, triggering the immune system to attack them. Pancreatic cancer vaccines are currently in the clinical trial phase. They are most often used in combination with chemotherapy and radiation to maximize their potential effect in shrinking tumors and prolonging patient life.

Johns Hopkins University began a clinical trial for a pancreatic cancer vaccine in 2001, and the study is continuing. Patients at Johns Hopkins who have had surgery for adenocarcinoma of the pancreas and who have no evidence of spread of the cancer outside of the pancreas may participate in the vaccine trial. Dr. Elizabeth Jaffee of Johns Hopkins originally developed the vaccine by culturing pancreatic tumor cells and introducing a protein called GM-CSF, which reproduces in cancer cells and helps to trigger the body's natural immune response once it is introduced via injection.

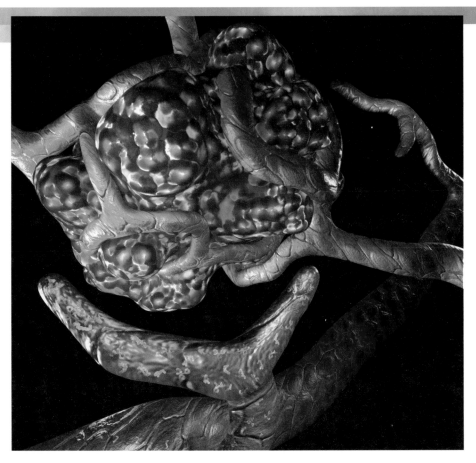

Bioengineered agents (green and yellow) are delivered through the bloodstream to the vessels feeding a tumor. These drugs will block new vessel growth and restrain or reverse the tumor's growth.

OTHER IMMUNE THERAPIES

Scientists are working to create monoclonal, or artificial, antibodies that they can inject into patients to stimulate the immune system. Monoclonal antibodies are created with an affinity for a specific molecule. One example is carcinoembryonic antigen (CEA), which is found on the surface of pancreatic cancer cells. Toxins or radioactive atoms can be attached to these antibodies, which are then carried directly to the tumor cells. Researchers hope that these lab-created antibodies will kill the cancer cells while ignoring normal, healthy cells nearby. This therapy is in the early development stage of clinical trials.

GENE THERAPY

In addition to vaccines, gene therapy for pancreatic cancer is also being carefully studied. The use of gene therapy to combat pancreatic cancer is still in its very early stages. Scientists around the world are beginning to develop reliable techniques to insert genes into cancer cells to fight the disease. At Johns Hopkins University, studies have identified a tumor suppressor gene, DCP4, which is missing or inactivated in more than half of all patients with pancreatic cancer. According to the researchers, "Losing the function of both pairs of this gene is similar to losing the brakes on a car, enabling the cancer cells to multiply unchecked." The team is currently investigating the possibility that inactivated tumor suppressor genes can be activated to destroy nearby cancer cells and combat the disease.

NEW DRUG THERAPIES

Nearly all medications are derived from carbon-based molecules, just as our human bodies are. However, in 2007, chemists at the University of Wisconsin-Madison replaced a carbon molecule in an anti-inflammatory and anticancer drug called indomethacin with a silicon molecule. They

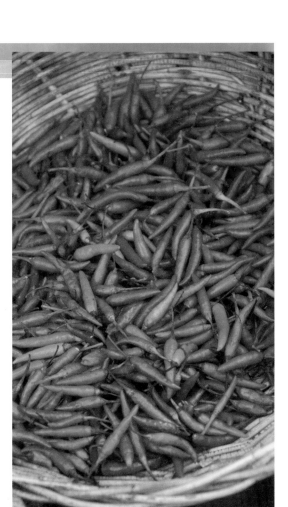

Capsaicin, the chemical compound that causes the "heat" in peppers, has been found to have a positive effect in fighting cancer, including pancreatic cancer.

found that it could be more effective in fighting cancers, particularly pancreatic cancer. Indomethacin was a drug with limited use in its traditional form because, though medically beneficial, it was also highly toxic. Tests are still under way to determine whether the new combination of silicon with this and other medications could prove to be effective against pancreatic and other cancers.

Natural compounds may also prove effective in the fight against pancreatic cancer. In 2006, researchers at the University of Pittsburgh School of Medicine conducted a series of studies in mice with pancreatic cancer and found that capsaicin—the ingredient that causes the "heat" in peppers—caused cancer growth to slow and tumors to shrink. Capsaicin caused the pancreatic cancer cells to die through a process called apoptosis. Apoptosis is the body's normal method of disposing of damaged or unneeded cells. It is often defective in cancer cells, and it is part of the reason that drug-resistant, fast-growing cancers like pancreatic cancer continue to thrive.

In May 2008, an herb used in traditional medicine in the Middle East was found to be beneficial in combating pancreatic cancer. Researchers at the Kimmel Cancer Center at Jefferson Medical College in Philadelphia, Pennsylvania, found that thymoquinone, a seed oil extract of the Middle Eastern herb *Nigella sativa*, blocked pancreatic cancer cell growth and killed the cells by enhancing the process of programmed cell death.

A HOPEFUL BUT UNPROVEN NEW THERAPY

Genes are the basic physical units of heredity in cells. They are specific sequences of bases that encode instructions on how to make proteins. Inside cells, proteins perform most of life's functions and are the primary components of cell structures. Genetic disorders can result from faulty expression of genes.

The most common form of gene therapy replaces a non-functional or malfunctioning gene with a normally functioning gene. Sometimes, abnormal genes can be repaired or regulated, rather than replaced. Gene therapy is not currently approved by the U.S. Food and Drug Administration (FDA) for patient treatment. Public attention was first drawn to gene therapy in 1999, when eighteen-year-old Jesse Gelsinger was undergoing a gene therapy trial for a hereditary illness. He died four days after starting the treatment, and his death was believed to have been triggered by a severe immune response to the viral carrier that administered the gene therapy treatment.

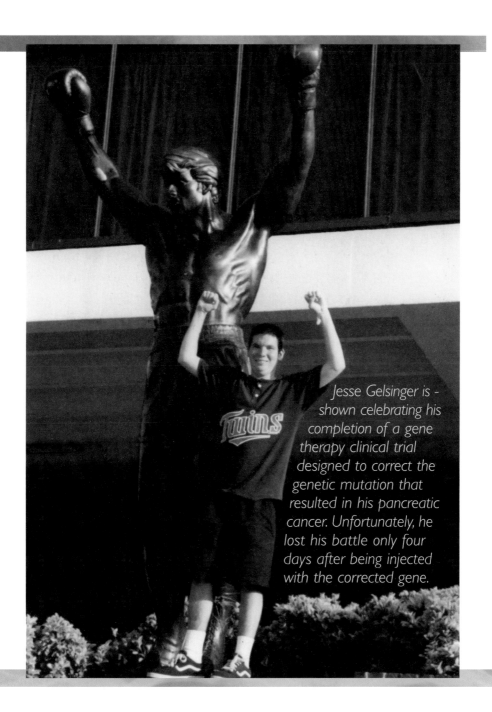

Jesse Gelsinger is - shown celebrating his completion of a gene therapy clinical trial designed to correct the genetic mutation that resulted in his pancreatic cancer. Unfortunately, he lost his battle only four days after being injected with the corrected gene.

THE HUMAN ELEMENT

In all medical research, the human element cannot be forgotten. Not only is pancreatic cancer a chilling diagnosis for patients to receive, it is also among the most painful and debilitating of cancers. Extreme weight loss or anorexia is common. Changes in the body's gastrointestinal system mean that patients cannot properly digest meals. The combination of chemotherapy and radiation can cause side effects ranging from severe nausea and exhaustion to hair loss and skin problems. Depression is common in cancer patients, making them more exhausted, anxious, and debilitated.

Dr. Dennis Lee was a Southern California physician and founder of Medicinenet.com, an online resource for patients and physicians. He had no risk factors for pancreatic cancer, yet he received an astonishing diagnosis of the disease in May 2007. Lee chronicled his cancer fight on Medicinenet.com. His cancer was inoperable when it was discovered—it had already spread to his liver.

Receiving a combination of chemotherapy and radiation, Lee's worst side effect was a sore mouth. Even though he lost weight, he still felt well enough to play tennis and attend a symposium sponsored by PanCAN, a pancreatic research support organization in Southern California. At the symposium, he met a number of pancreatic cancer survivors, which showed him that the diagnosis was not universally fatal.

Lee wrote in March 2008 that "all my journal readings and past experiences as a doctor tell me that my prognosis is poor. But let me share with you a small secret: In tennis terms, I believe the match is going to be decided by a long tiebreaker in the fifth set, and I am afraid I will win this one."

Sadly, Lee's prediction did not come true. He lost his battle with pancreatic cancer on April 11, 2008.

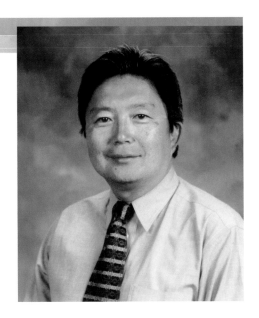

Pictured here is Dr. Dennis Lee. Lee, a prominent physician and founder of Medicinenet.com, lost his battle with pancreatic cancer on April 11, 2008.

It is hoped that by continuing the fight—through research and the development of new treatments and clinical trials in gene therapy and cancer vaccines—pancreatic cancer can move from being one of the most fatal of cancers to becoming one of the most curable. Early diagnosis and detection are key. Pancreatic cancer's status as the "silent killer" and its difficulty in diagnosing early have been the main barriers to successful treatment in the past. With recent increases in funding and research, the frightening diagnosis of pancreatic cancer may soon become less so. Pancreatic cancer may become not only a disease than can be managed and fought, but also one that can be cured or even prevented altogether.

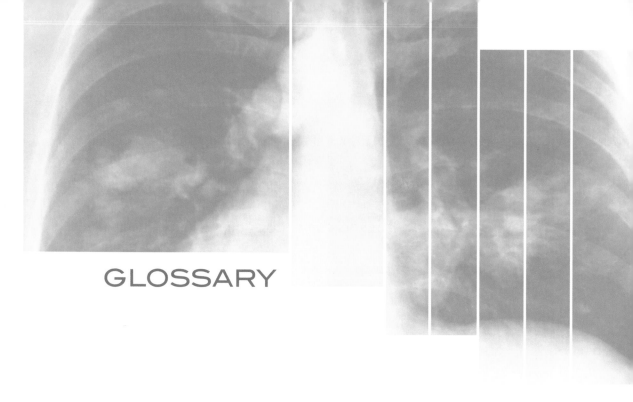

GLOSSARY

adenocarcinoma A cancer that develops in the cells lining glandular internal organs, including the lungs, breasts, ovaries, colon, prostate, and pancreas.

adjuvant therapy Secondary treatment given after the primary treatment (usually surgery) to increase the chances of a cure. Adjuvant therapy may include chemotherapy, radiation therapy, hormone therapy, or biological therapy.

biopsy The medical removal of cells or body tissue for examination, testing, and diagnosis.

clinical trial A formal medical research process to determine the safety and effectiveness of medical procedures or medications.

duct A passage in the body carrying glandular fluid, including bile and other digestive enzymes.

endocrine glands Glands in the body that produce hormones that are usually released directly into the bloodstream and that can affect a wide variety of body functions. The pancreas contains both endocrine and exocrine cells.

endoscopic Looking inside the body without surgery.

exocrine pancreas Cells within the pancreas that release enzymes through a duct system, which carries the enzymes through the rest of the body. The pancreas secretes digestive enzymes through its ducts that feed into the small intestine.

gene therapy Medical treatments that involve the manipulation and use of genetic material.

inoperable The medical term for a cancer or other condition that cannot be treated surgically.

jaundice A condition caused by blockage of bile ducts from the liver that causes the digestive fluid bile to accumulate, leading to yellow eyes and skin.

metastatic cancer Cancer that begins in one organ and then spreads to other locations in the body.

oncogene A gene capable, when activated, of transforming a cell and causing cancer.

primary cancer A tumor arising in the first organ it affects.

resectable A medical term for a cancer or other tumor or foreign body that can be surgically removed or treated effectively by surgery.

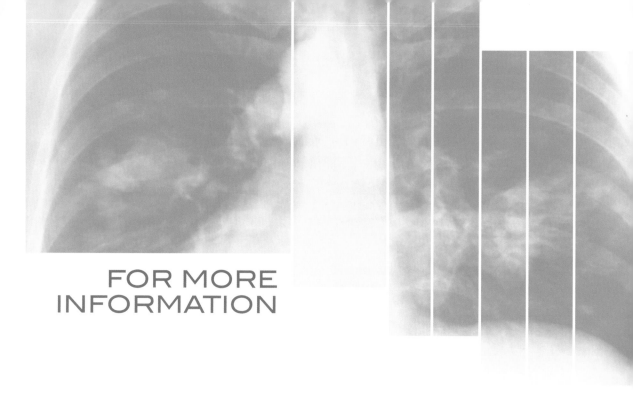

FOR MORE INFORMATION

Canadian Cancer Society
10 Alcorn Avenue, Suite 200
Toronto, ON M4V 3B1
Canada
(416) 961-7223
Web site: http://www.cancer.ca
The Canadian Cancer Society supports research and provides education, support, and other programs, including prevention and care, for cancer patients, members of the general public, physicians, and caregivers.

Hirshberg Foundation for Pancreatic Research
2990 South Sepulveda Boulevard, Suite 300C
Los Angeles, CA 90064
(310) 473-5121
Web site: http://www.pancreatic.org
The Hirshberg Foundation raises funds for pancreatic research and supports the Hirshberg Center for Pancreatic Cancer at the

University of California, Los Angeles. Resources for patients and support groups are available.

Lustgarten Foundation for Pancreatic Cancer Research
1111 Stewart Avenue
Bethpage, NY 11714
(516) 803-2304
Web site: http://www.lustgarten.org
The Lustgarten Foundation funds clinical research into pancreatic cancer and provides resources for patients and caregivers. It also sponsors a clinical trials matching service for patients with pancreatic cancer.

PanCAN: Pancreatic Cancer Action Network
2141 Rosecrans Avenue, Suite 7000
El Segundo, CA 90245
(877) 272-6226 (toll free); (310) 725-0025
Web site: http://www.pancan.org
PanCAN funds many different forms of pancreatic research and supports patient registries that can help family members as well as direct future research.

WEB SITES
Due to the changing nature of Internet links, Rosen Publishing has developed an online list of Web sites related to the subject of this book. This site is updated regularly. Please use this link to access this list:

http://www.rosenlinks.com/cms/panc

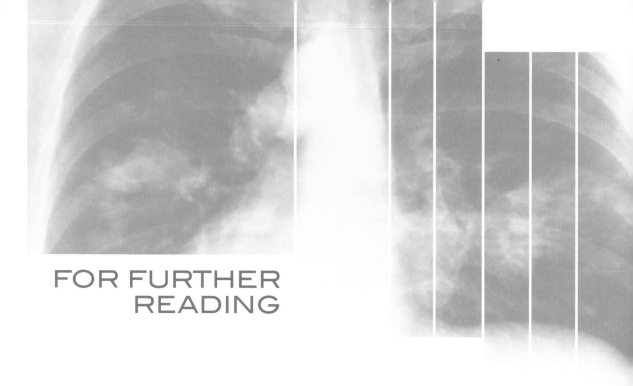

FOR FURTHER READING

Buckingham, Dorothea. *Staring Down the Dragon*. Leland, NC: Sydney Press, 2007.

Davis, Devra. *The Secret History of the War on Cancer*. New York, NY: Basic Books, 2007.

DiGiacomo, Fran. *I'd Rather Do Chemo Than Clean Out the Garage*. Dallas, TX: Brown Books, 2003.

Dreyer, Zoann. *Living with Cancer* (Teen's Guides). New York, NY: Facts On File, 2008.

Mareck, Amy M. *Fighting for My Life: Growing Up with Cancer*. Minneapolis, MN: Fairview Press, 2007.

Panno, Joseph. *Gene Therapy: Treating Disease by Repairing Genes*. New York, NY: Facts On File, 2004.

Pausch, Randy. *The Last Lecture*. New York, NY: Hyperion, 2008.

Rains, Calvin G., Sr. *My Journey with Pancreatic Cancer*. Bloomington, IN: AuthorHouse, 2006.

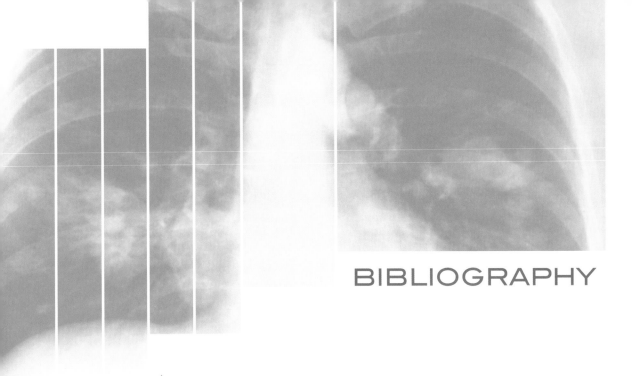

BIBLIOGRAPHY

American Cancer Society. "Cancer Statistics 2008 Presentation." 2008. Retrieved March 22, 2008 (http://www.cancer.org/docroot/PRO/content/PRO_1_1_Cancer_Statistics_2008_Presentation.asp).

American Cancer Society. "What Is Pancreatic Cancer?" June 8, 2008. Retrieved March 13, 2008 (http://www.cancer.org/docroot/CRI/content/CRI_2_2_1X_What_is_pancreatic_cancer_34.asp?rnav=cri).

Cameron, John L. *Pancreatic Cancer* (American Cancer Society Atlas of Clinical Oncology). Hamilton, ON, Canada: BC Decker, 2001.

Devitt, Terry. "Silicon Medicines May Be Effective in Humans." *University of Wisconsin-Madison News*, January 24, 2007. Retrieved March 22, 2008 (http://www.news.wisc.edu/13376).

Grady, Denise. "In a Former First Family, Cancer Has a Grim Legacy." *New York Times*, August 7, 2007. Retrieved March 13, 2008 (http://www.nytimes.com/2007/08/07/health/07jimm.html?_r=1&oref=slogin).

Human Genome Project Information. "Gene Therapy." March 13, 2008. Retrieved March 19, 2008 (http://www.ornl.gov/sci/techresources/Human_Genome/medicine/genetherapy.shtml#whatis).

Johns Hopkins Medicine: The Sol Goldman Pancreatic Research Center. "The Genetics of Pancreatic Cancer—The Discoveries—K-ras Mutations." January 20, 2004. Retrieved March 13, 2008 (http://pathology2.jhu.edu/PANCREAS/geneticsweb/K-ras.htm).

Johns Hopkins Medicine: The Sol Goldman Pancreatic Research Center. "The National Familial Pancreatic Cancer Registry." August 1, 2007. Retrieved March 20, 2008 (http://pathology.jhu.edu/pancreas/PartNFPTR.php).

Kim, Y. K. R. "The Mouse in Science: Cancer Research." University of California Davis Center for Animal Alternatives, 1996. Retrieved March 18, 2008 (http://www.vetmed.ucdavis.edu/Animal_Alternatives/cancer.htm).

Lee, Dennis. "Pancreatic Cancer, the Silent Disease." Medicinenet.com, April 18, 2008. Retrieved April 20, 2008 (http://www.medicinenet.com/script/main/art.asp?articlekey=84931).

Leonard, Leslie. "Nanotechnology and Pancreatic Cancer." Johns Hopkins Medicine, 2005. Retrieved March 18, 2008 (http://pathology.jhu.edu/pancreas/presentations.php?area=nu#).

Loft, Maxwell A. *Trends in Pancreatic Cancer Research*. New York, NY: Nova Biomedical Books, 2005.

National Cancer Institute. "Cancer Research Portfolio—Pancreatic Cancer Project List." 2008. Retrieved March 20, 2008 (http://researchportfolio.cancer.gov/projectlist.jsp?result=true&strSearchID=325122&strApp=CRP).

National Cancer Institute. "Pancreatic Cancer: Six Years of Research Progress." December 2007. Retrieved March 13, 2008 (http://planning.cancer.gov/disease/2007PancreaticProgRpt.pdf).

O'Malley, Lauren. "New Information About the Precursors to Pancreatic Cancer." Johns Hopkins Medicine, 2006. Retrieved March 18, 2008 (http://pathology.jhu.edu/pancreas/presentations.php?area=nu#).

O'Reilly, Eileen. *100 Questions About Pancreatic Cancer.* Sudbury, MA: Jones & Bartlett, 2002.

Riess, H., et al., eds. *Pancreatic Cancer* (Recent Results in Cancer Research). New York, NY: Springer, 2007.

Science Daily. "Traditional Herbal Medicine Kills Pancreatic Cancer, Researchers Report." May 20, 2008. Retrieved May 20, 2008 (http://www.sciencedaily.com/releases/2008/05/080519092215.htm).

Science News. "Anti-inflammatory Prevents Pancreatic Cancer in Mice." August 18, 2007. Retrieved March 15, 2008 (http://find.galegroup.com/itx/start.do?prodId=EAIM).

Szabo, Liz. "The Monster in the Family." *USA Today,* June 12, 2005. Retrieved March 15, 2008 (http://www.usatoday.com/news/health/2005-06-12-pancreatic-cover_x.htm).

VonHoff, Daniel D. *Pancreatic Cancer.* Sudbury, MA: Jones & Bartlett, 2005.

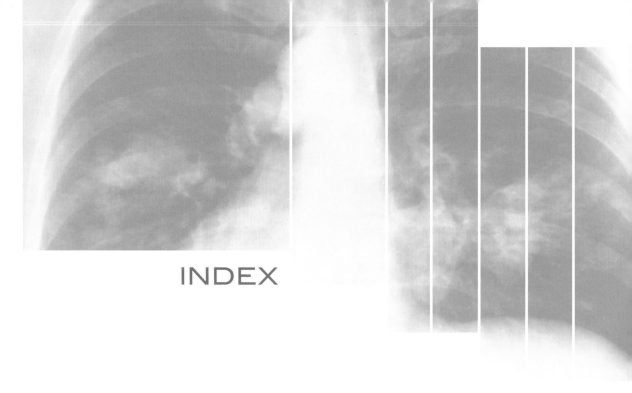

INDEX

ABOUT THE AUTHOR

Amy Sterling Casil is an award-nominated writer, and her subjects have frequently involved future trends in medicine and biology. A fifth-generation Southern California native, she has published eighteen books, including several written for the Rosen Publishing Group. She lives in Redlands, California, with her daughter, a high school student. Her personal experience with pancreatic cancer contributed to the writing of this book. Her mother, Sterling Sturtevant, an Academy Award–winning art director of animated films, died of pancreatic cancer at age forty.

PHOTO CREDITS